Bericht aus dem Nationalen Referenzlabor des BVL für das Jahr 2008

Technical Report on the Activities of the Community Reference Laboratory for Residues of β-Agonists, Coccidiostats, Anthelmintics and NSAIDs for the Period 1 January to 31 December 2008

Contents

General		5
1	General tasks	6
	1.1 Meeting 4 CRLs; EC-4 CRL for residues management	6
	1.2 EC/CRL related EC and International Bodies; Co-operation with international organisations	6
	1.3 Reports, cost estimate, documentation	7
2	Development and validation of analytical methods	8
	2.1 Investigation of distribution/depletion of nitroimidazoles in hens	8
	2.2 Development and validation of a method for 29 beta agonists in hair and urine by LC-MS/MS	12
	2.3 Validation of method for 29 beta-agonists in retina by LC-MSMS	13
	2.4 Optimisation and validation of method for 5 avermectins in aquaculture products	15
	2.5 Long term stability studies for all substance groups	16
	2.6 Research and identification of new or unknown compounds	18
3	Quality assurance and quality control including the development of incurred test material and the organisation of a proficiency test	19
	3.1 Maintenance of equipment, documentation, audits, management	19
	3.2 Proficiency test on benzimidazoles in milk: characterisation of the material, packaging, evaluation	19
	3.3 Cooperation with IRMM for the production of CRM for nitroimidazoles	20
	3.4 Production of incurred sample material	20
4	Technical and scientific support to Member States and the Commission including arbitration and training activities	22
	4.1 Technical, scientific support and training	22
	4.2 Follow-up of proficiency test	22
	4.3 Provision of standard substances, reference materials and methods incl. procuring, storage, administration, documentation, shipment etc.	22
	4.4 Analysis of official samples	24
	4.5 Visit to NRLs	24
	4.6 Organisation and realisation of a Workshop: measurement uncertainty, analytical news and problems	25
	4.7 Publications, reports and contributions	25
	4.8 Presentations	26
	4.9 Staff of the CRL Berlin	26
	4.10 Organigram of the CRL Berlin	27
5	Breakdown of personel and financial capacities (Annex)	28

General

The European Community Reference Laboratory for residues of beta-agonists, anticoccidials including nitroimidazoles, anthelmintics and non-steroidal anti-inflammatory drugs (NSAIDs) at the BVL *(Bundesamt für Verbraucherschutz und Lebensmittelsicherheit)* is part of Group 5 "Analyses" (cf. organigram in chapter 5). The CRL is represented by unit 502 which is also the NRL for the substance groups the CRL is responsible for.

The analytical activities of the CRL Berlin are pursued by two specialised sub-units, one being responsible for GC and GC-MS, one for HPLC and LC-MS. They are supplemented by a third sub-unit in charge of the preparation of incurred test materials to be used as in-house reference samples and for proficiency testing.

The activities listed in the following correspond to the duties and operating conditions of CRLs as laid down in Annex V, Chapter 2 of Council Directive 96/23/EC of 29 April 1996. The respective sections of Council Directive 96/23/EC are indicated at the beginning of each chapter.

1 General tasks

1.1
Meeting 4 CRLs; EC-4 CRL for residues management

The coordination meeting of the four CRLs for residues was substituted by a meeting at the EuroResidue Conference VI, Egmond aan Zee, The Netherlands, on 20 May 2008.

During the meeting the focus of the discussion was laid upon the question of how to proceed with the draft guideline on the validation of screening methods and the question of how to assess positive findings of substances for which a sum MRL has been established.

1.2
EC/CRL related EC and International Bodies; Co-operation with international organisations

The CRL was asked for and issued statements on reports of the CCMAS working group, especially on questions concerning the establishment of criteria for single laboratory validation and recovery correction, settling of disputes and measurement uncertainty. Statements of the German delegation were sent to the EU codex secretariat via the German ministry for consumer protection, food and agriculture (BMVEL).

With respect to traceability and comparability questions the CRL is still in contact with the Physikalisch-Technische Bundesanstalt (PTB) in Braunschweig, Germany (the National Metrology Institute of Germany). A contract for an official cooperation was issued and signed in 2004 with the aim to attain a designation of the BVL-CRL/NRL as laboratory measuring with highest precision and accuracy. In February 2008 the CRL/NRL for residues was nominated as designated institute to fulfil the tasks of a National Metrology Institute, NMI, by the PTB, which was acknowledged by the BIPM (international Bureau of Weights and Measures). In this context a report was issued on the pilot study performed in 2007 and presented at the CCQM (Consultative Committee for Amount of Substance) meeting in Paris in April 2008. The head of the CRL Berlin participated in the OAWG (organic analysis working group) of CCQM from 31 March to 01 April 2008.

As a member of the ISO/CEN TC 34 SC 9 WG 3 on "Validation of microbiological procedures" the head of the CRL participated in WG 3 meetings twice, on 16 and 17 January in London and on 29 and 30 September in Bergamo/Italy. In this context the national mirror group meetings were visited and a concept for the alternative validation of microbiological methods was developed and presented and discussed at the ISO/CEN WG 3 meetings and at the national meetings.

The CRL provided support to the respective Commission services regarding the following topics:
- Participation in a one-week FVO mission to Spain in March 2008 as national expert,
- Validation: supportive information on the validation of screening methods to the CRL Fougères as well as to DG SANCO, unit E3,
- Codex Alimentarius (CCMAS): provision of statements on CCMAS papers for the European secretariat,
- Evaluation of the MS residue control plans of 2008 in connection with the results of 2007 to provide recommendations for improvements,
- Participation in a DG SANCO meeting on residue control plans in June 2008,
- Participation in the EuroResidue Conference in May 2008 including the presentation of 11 posters, 3 oral presentations and chairing the workshop "update on legislation, a. o. validation of bioassays, measurement uncertainty",
- Cooperation with IRMM in the preparation of CRM for nitroimidazoles. The CRL is performing all investigations on the commutability of the matrices and techniques,
- Participation in a CAP (Commission Advisory Panel for small organic molecules) meeting of IRMM, Geel, in April, September and November 2008, in the framework of the production of certified reference material,
- Participation in a meeting on ractopamine of the EFSA Panel on Additives and Products used in Animal Feed (FEEDAP), 17 Dec. 2008,
- Ongoing elaboration of a concept for the validation of microbiological and immunological screening methods,
- Ongoing elaboration of a concept of how to assess positive findings of substances which have sum MRL (problem of decision making and calculation of measurement uncertainty). The final document could be published in December 2008 and is available at the CRL website: http://fis-vl.bund.de/Public/irc/fis-vl/Home/main?index,
- Assessment of Codex MRL concerning veterinary drugs,
- Information in form of publications and own studies on ractopamine was provided with respect to toxicity, distribution in the animal, depletion times etc.

1.3
Reports, cost estimate, documentation

The CRL management drew up a cost estimate and a work plan for the next contract period from 1 January to 31 December 2009. In this context the new regulations as laid down in Commission Regulation 1754/2006 have to be respected, which also apply for the budgeting of the forthcoming workshop. Additionally, the report on the reference period January to December 2007 and the interim report for 2008 were prepared. The report on the CRL-workshop was submitted as well.

2 Development and validation of analytical methods[1]

2.1 Investigation of distribution/depletion of nitroimidazoles in hens

Groups of 3 hens each were formed and one drug per group was applied (ronidazole, metronidazole, tinidazole and carnidazole, respectively). The drugs were applied via the drinking water with an estimated dosage of 10 mg/kg body weight and day. The hens were treated for 5 days; 24 h before slaughtering the medication was discontinued. The samples were collected directly after slaughtering. The muscle samples were taken in two different ways: i) portioned and directly deep-frozen; ii) portioned, stored at RT for 2 h, then stored overnight at +4 °C (18 h) and transferred to –25 °C the next day. The procedure ii) was chosen in order to simulate less careful/inadequate sampling conditions.

2.1.1 Studies on stability and homogeneity in muscle

Due to the limited amount of incurred matrix material available from hens, a combined approach for the tests on homogeneity and stability was chosen. Identical looking pieces of muscle of approximately 100 g were taken for each of the sampling procedures (see above) from metronidazole- and ronidazole-treated animals. The muscle was cut into sub-samples of approximately 15–20 g. Each of the sub-samples was analysed in triplicate (analytical sample: 4 g). The results are shown in the *Fig. 2-1*. Black rhombi represent the values for muscle directly frozen (–25 °C) after slaughtering and packaging; light grey squares represent the values for muscle of the same kind and same animal but stored overnight at +4 °C before deep-freezing. The big symbols show the mean values of the triplicate determinations of the individual pieces of muscle and the small symbols indicate the single values in order to show the distribution of the measurement values.

The distribution of the single measurements clearly indicates that the analytes are distributed inhomogeneously in the matrix muscle – this is true for the drug itself as well as for the corresponding metabolite. Partly the concentrations vary by a factor of two or more between the three determinations.

Furthermore it becomes obvious that a less careful sampling leads to a partly dramatic loss of analytes. E.g. in case of MNZ no residues at all could be detected when applying this sampling procedure. Since this is true also for the hydroxy-metabolite, it can be concluded that the loss of MNZ due to a metabolisation to MNZOH is unlikely, or the metabolite degrades as rapidly as the drug itself. In case of RNZ the drug as well as partly the hydroxy-metabolite can still be found, but in significantly lower concentrations.

The approach of combining the homogeneity and stability study directly with the slaughtering, without being biased by other processes, e.g. repeated thawing, proved to be very helpful.

2.1.2 Studies on stability and homogeneity in plasma/serum

The results for stability and homogeneity in plasma and partly in serum are presented in *Fig. 2-2*. The graphs compare the results determined in the plasma of MNZ- and RNZ-treated hens directly frozen after sampling to plasma which was stored for 1 week at +4 °C. For MNZ-treated animals, the results for serum are also included. Each of the samples was analysed in triplicate again. The CVs for the triplicate determinations are below 5%, indicating a good homogeneity of the samples. There is no significant difference between plasma frozen directly and after storage at +4 °C, and the serum shows comparable residue levels. Furthermore, the mean residue levels found in the corresponding muscle samples, which are significantly lower than the plasma/serum levels, are included in the figures.

2.1.3 Carnidazole- and tinidazole-treated animals

Even though the method has not yet been validated for these compounds, the quantification with matrix calibration curves yielded good results for spiked matrix samples (quality control samples). Hence, the method was applied to incurred samples. Examples of chromatograms of muscle samples are given in *Fig. 2-3* and *2-4*.

As far as it can be concluded from this limited set of data, the parent drugs can be found in muscle as well as in plasma. The highest levels are present in plasma, which also was the case for MNZ and RNZ. The concentration levels are 1–2 µg/kg for CNZ

---
[1] Annex V, chapter 2, section 1 (a, c, d)

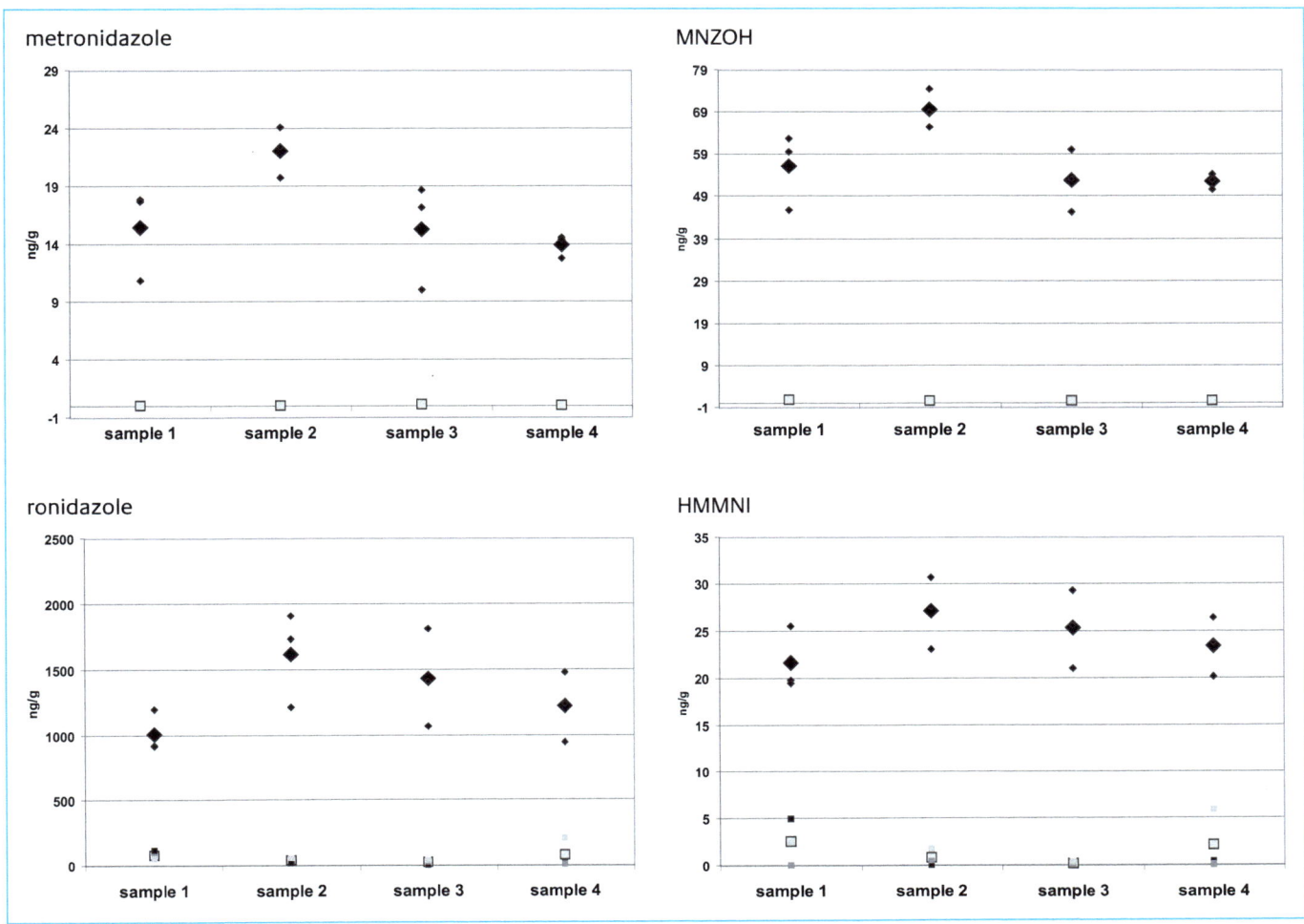

Fig. 2-1 Results of the combined homogeneity/stability study for hens muscle (further details in the text).

and TIZ in muscle and 2–5 µg/kg in plasma. This suggests that these compounds cause lower residue levels than MNZ or especially RNZ – presuming that all animals received the same drug dosages. On the other hand, it has to be taken into account that the level of nitroimidazole residues found in the three animals within one group may vary considerably in parts. This may be due to two reasons: natural biovariability or a different drug intake/withdrawal period. The exact intake could not be controlled since the drugs were administered in drinking water. A final decision on the share of the two possible contributions to the final effect cannot be made with this experimental design.

2.1.4 Metabolisation and hydroxy-metabolites

As it was the case for pigs, the hydroxy-metabolite is the dominant residue in MNZ-treated animals, while for ronidazole, it is by far the drug itself. The ratio of drug to metabolite is similar in all matrices for RNZ and HMMNI. For MNZ, the hydroxy-metabolite is present in higher ratios in plasma than in muscle.

For carnidazole and tinidazole the sample extracts were checked for the possible presence of hydroxy-metabolites ($C_8H_{12}N_4O_4S$ and $C_8H_{13}N_3O_5S$, respectively) in preliminary measurements with a Q-TOF system (Agilent LC 1200 / QTOF 6520, full scan mode, exact mass measurement with a resolution of >10,000). Only in case of tinidazole signals of potential oxidation products were found. There were two peaks, which could refer to oxidation products with an intact ring structure. This would be in agreement with the findings made for the tinidazole metabolism in humans, where two hydroxy-metabolites (2-hydroxymethyl-tinidazole and 1-(2-ethylsulfonylethyl)-5-hydroxy-2-methyl-4-nitroimidazole) were identified. In order to prove the identity of the peaks it is planned to synthesize the supposed compounds for use as reference. However, this process has not been finalised yet.

2.1.5 Stability and metabolisation in egg samples

Hens were treated with different nitroimidazoles for 2–3 weeks. Nitroimidazole residues could be detected up to 7 days after withdrawal of the drug. The analytes themselves proved to be stable in mixed fresh egg for at least one week when stored at +4 °C. With respect to metabolisation, the hydroxy-metabolite

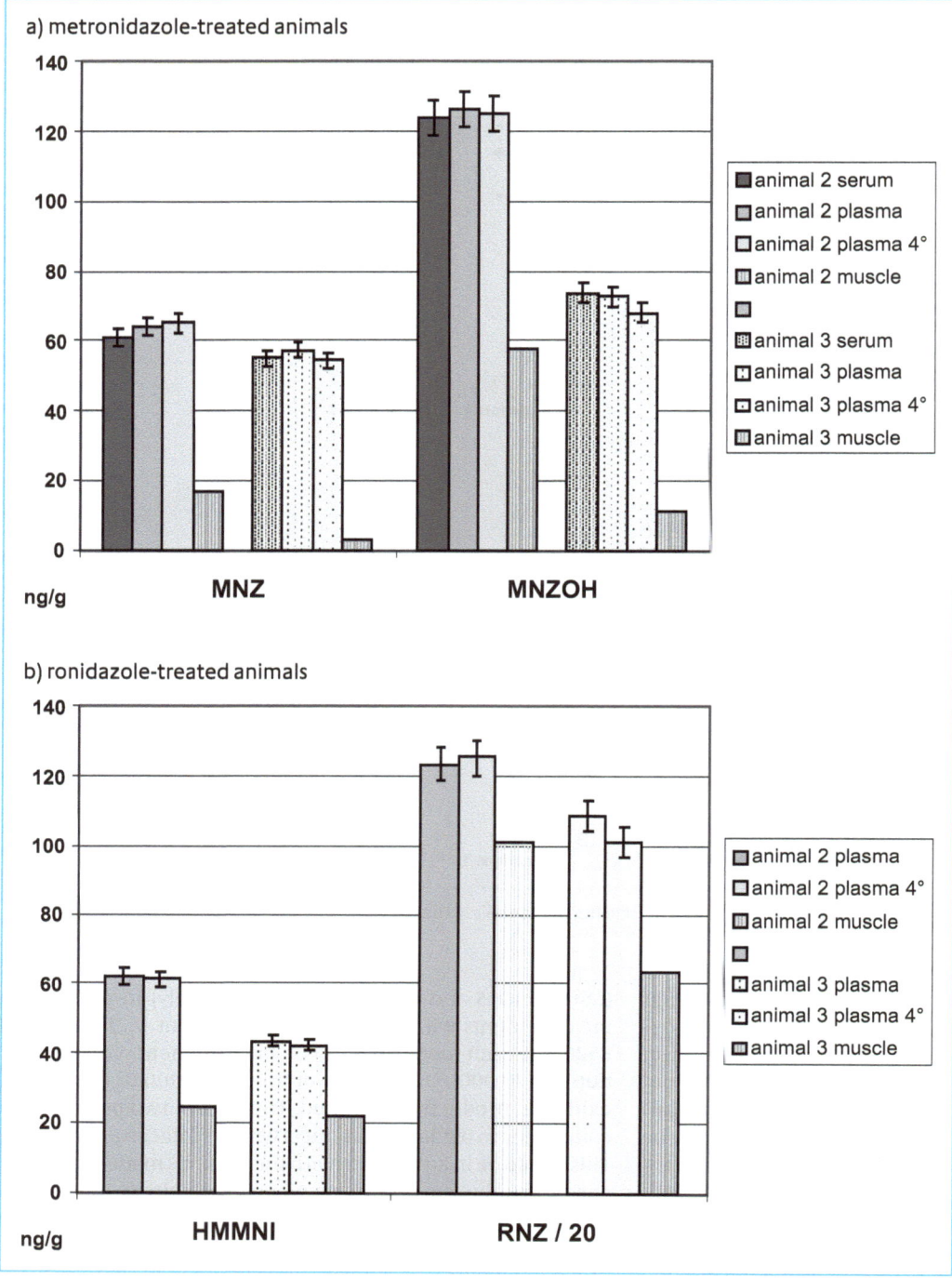

Fig. 2-2 Comparison of nitroimidazole residues in plasma, in plasma stored for 1 week at +4 °C, in serum and in muscle (further details in the text).

HMMNI was the dominant residue in eggs of dimetridazole-treated hens (DMZ approx. 10–20% of HMMNI) and IPZOH was the dominant residue in ipronidazole-treated hens (IPZ approx. 2–10% of IPZOH). For ronidazole, the drug itself was the dominant residue (HMMNI < 5% of RNZ), while for metronidazole the situation changed after the withdrawal of the drug: during the application of metronidazole, the drug itself was dominant (ratio MNZ/MNZOH approx. 2:1), while in the course of the withdrawal of the drug, MNZOH became the dominant residue. After 7 days of withdrawal, only MNZOH was detected.

2.1.6 Summary

Based on the results of the present studies, earlier studies with turkeys and in-house studies for the production of reference materials and proficiency tests, the following conclusions can be drawn with regard to an effective residue control.

Depending on the matrix/species, nitroimidazoles tend to degrade in matrix, hence special care has to be taken regarding sampling, sample storage and analytical conditions.

Plasma or retina should be the preferred matrices for resi-

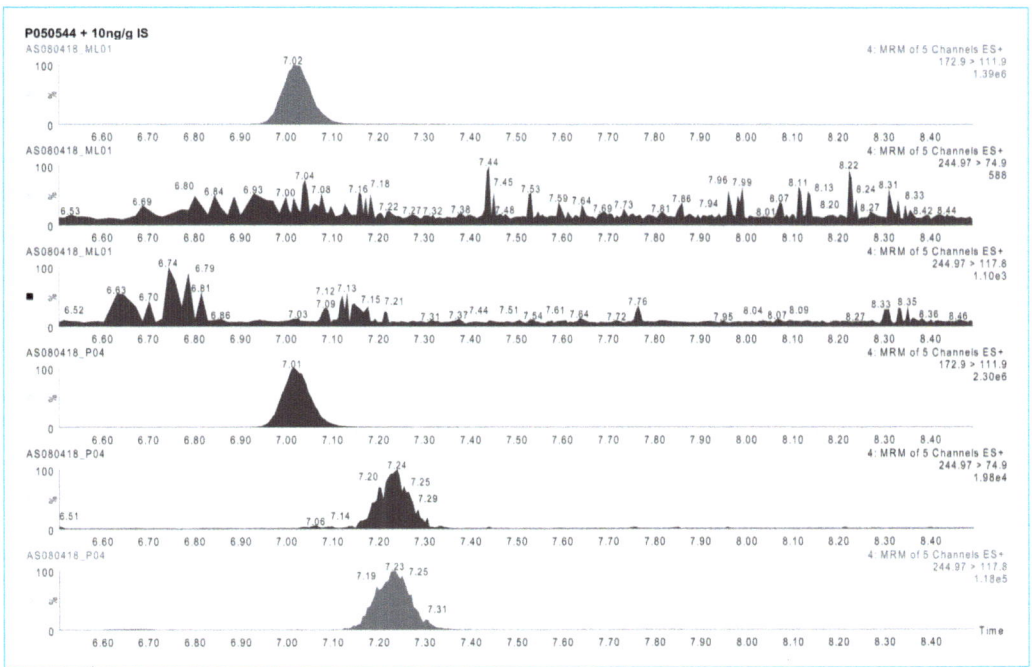

Fig. 2-3 Example of an incurred muscle sample of carnidazole (1 ng/g); ion traces 1–3: blank matrix (ion trace 1: internal standard D3-IPZ at 10 ng/g); ion traces 4–6: incurred muscle (ion trace 4: internal standard D3-IPZ at 10 ng/g).

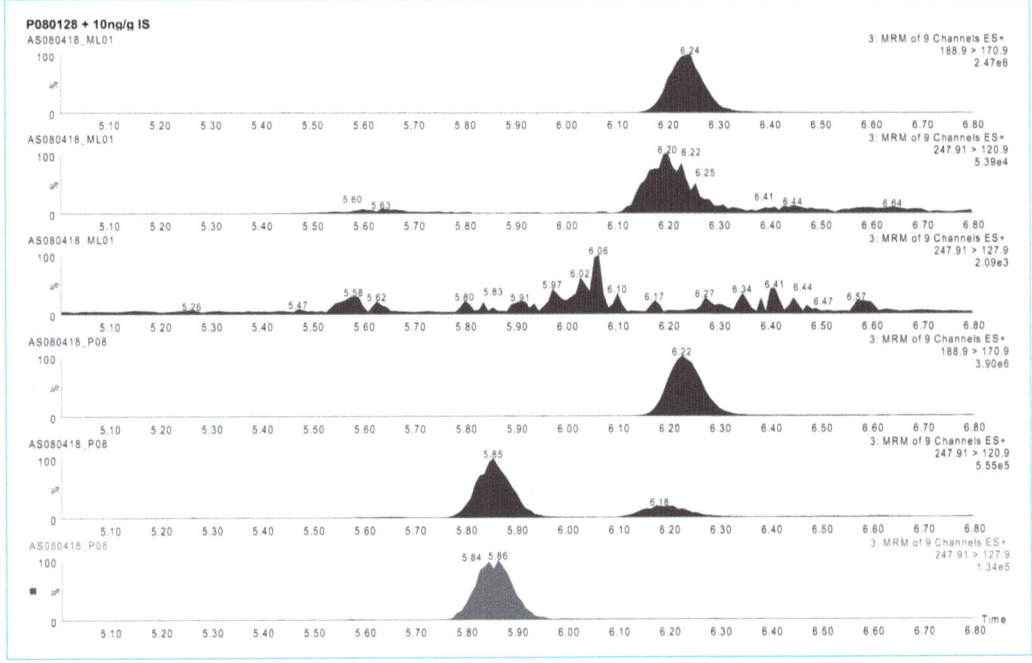

Fig. 2-4 Example of an incurred muscle sample of tinidazole (2 ng/g); ion traces 1–3: blank matrix (ion trace 1: internal standard D3-IPZOH at 10 ng/g); ion traces 4–6: incurred muscle (ion trace 4: internal standard D3-IPZOH at 10 ng/g).

due control. For the matrix muscle a homogenous distribution cannot be presumed, hence problems may arise with respect to the comparability of results, e.g. in case of counter-analyses by different laboratories.

The general ratio of drug to hydroxy-metabolite was similar in all species. DMZ and IPZ metabolize rapidly, consequently the hydroxy-metabolite is the main residue. For RNZ the drug itself is the main residue. MNZ and its hydroxy-metabolite lie in between, i.e. partly the drug, partly the hydroxy-metabolite is dominant. Since the studies showed that the ratio of drug to hydroxy-metabolite is not constant throughout the withdrawal period, it is always recommendable to control the drug as well as the hydroxy-metabolite.

A carnidazole and tinidazole medication of animals can be detected by the analysis of the parent drugs.

2.2 Development and validation of a method for 29 beta agonists in hair and urine by LC-MS/MS

2.2.1 Hair

A method for the determination of β-agonists in hair was developed and prepared for validation. The validation of the method started with 29 β-agonists. The results of validation for three substances (orciprenaline, pirbuterol and carbuterol) were not in accordance with the criteria of the Commission Decision 2002/657/EC. For that reason these analytes were not included in the summary of validation parameters.

The method is suitable for the identification and quantification of the following 26 β-agonists in hair: Bamethan, Brombuterol, Bromchlorbuterol, Carbuterol, Cimaterol, Cimbuterol, Clenbuterol, Clencyclohexerol, Clenhexerol, Clenisopenterol, Clenpenterol, Clenproperol, Hydroxy-methylclenbuterol, Fenoterol, Formoterol, Isoxsuprine, Labetalol, Mabuterol, Mapenterol, Ractopamine, Ritodrine, Salbutamol, Salmeterol, Sotalol, Terbutaline, Tulobuterol, Zilpaterol.

The following deuterated compounds were used as internal standards: Cimaterol-d7, Cimbuterol-d9, Clenbuterol-d9, Clenproperol-d7, Isoxsuprine-d5, Ractopamine-d5, Salbutamol-d9, Salmeterol-d3, Mabuterol-d9, Mapenterol-d11.

Principle of the method:
⇒ 1 g of hair is washed with 5–10 ml of 0.1 M hydrochloric acid in ethanol
⇒ Filtration
⇒ The hair is dried at 80 °C in a drying oven
⇒ Homogenisation of the hair in a ball mill
⇒ Samples of 100 mg are taken and extracted for 4 hours at 40 °C in an ultrasonic bath
⇒ After centrifugation internal standards are added to the extract and evaporated to dryness
⇒ The residue is re-dissolved in 10 ml of phosphate buffer, pH 6
⇒ The extract is purified by means of SPE using CleanScreen cartridges
⇒ The measurement is performed with LC-MS/MS

HPLC Parameters
- Column: Phenomenex LUNA C18, 150 × 2 mm, 3 µ
- Column temp.: 40 °C
- Flow: 300 µl/min
- Mobile phase A: 0.05 M ammonium formate in water, pH 4
- Mobile phase B: acetonitrile/0.05 M ammonium formate in water, pH 4 = 95:5
- Gradient: 0.00–3 min 90% A, within 7 min to 85% A, within 15 min to 60% A, within 3 min to 40% A, within 1 min to 90% A, 9 min at 90% A
- Injection volume: 20 µl
- Detection: MRM mode using ESI+ ionisation

2.2.2 Urine

In the CRL-Berlin a multi-method for confirmation and quantization of β-agonists in urine was validated on an API4000 triple quad MS few years ago. The aim was to extend this validation to other triple quad MS instruments with different instrument characteristics: a Waters Quattro Premier XE system coupled with an UPLC instead of HPLC and an API2000 system coupled with "normal" HPLC. Whereas the sensitivity of the API2000 system is lower than the API4000, the Premier XE system offers a similar sensitivity but exhibits due to use of UPLC shorter run times and increased chromatographic resolution. In order to check the applicability of the two alternative mass spectrometers for determination β-agonists in urine the repeatability of the instruments and the lowest concentration level which can be confirmed were investigated.

The following overview gives the instrument parameters of the different systems:

Applied Biosystem API 4000/Agilent HP 1100
HPLC (Agilent HP 1100)
- Column: Phenomenex LUNA C18, 150 × 2 mm, 3 µ
- Column temp.: 40 °C
- Flow: 300 µl/min
- Mobile phase A: 0.05 M ammonium formate in water, pH 4
- Mobile phase B: acetonitrile/0.05 M ammonium formate in water, pH 4 = 95:5
- Gradient: 0.00–3 min 90% A, within 7 min to 85% A, within 15 min to 60% A, within 3 min to 40% A, within 1 min to 90% A, 9 min at 90% A
- Injection volume: 20 µl

Triple mass spectrometer (API4000, Applied Biosystems)
- Source Temp.: 500 °C
- Ionisation: 5500 V
- CAD-gas: 6.0
- CUR-gas: 40.0
- Gas 1: 40.0
- Gas 2: 60.0

Applied Biosystem API 2000/Agilent HP 1100
HPLC (Agilent HP1100)
- Same as for API4000

Triple mass spectrometer (API2000, Applied Biosystems)
- Source Temp.: 450 °C
- Ionisation: 5500 V
- CAD-gas: 7.0
- CUR-gas: 25.0
- Gas 1: 30.0
- Gas 2: 80.0

Tab. 2-1 Comparison of the lowest concentration which can be confirmed if an API2000 system or a Quattro Premier XE systems is used. The resulting levels are compared with the CCα of the full validation on API400.

Analyte	API 4000* CCα [µg/kg]	API 2000 [µg/kg]	Premier XE [µg/kg]
Bamethan	1.12	2.12	1.51
Brombuterol	0.081	0.29	0.17
Bromchlorbuterol	0.040	0.21	0.08
Carbuterol	0.43	5.14	0.52
Cimaterol	0.15	0.35	0.18
Cimbuterol	0.073	0.27	0.15
Clenbuterol	0.035	0.26	0.09
Clencyclohexerol	0.16	0.51	0.34
Clenhexerol	0.18	0.51	0.56
Clenisopenterol	0.15	0.35	0.23
Clenpenterol	0.17	0.34	0.26
Clenproperol	0.09	0.39	0.16
Hydroxymethyl-clenb.	0.087	0.28	0.15
Fenoterol	0.41	4.65	0.44
Formoterol	1.01	1.09	0.99
Isoxsuprine	0.077	0.22	0.11
Labetalol	1.12	1.67	1.11
Mabuterol	0.031	0.19	0.06
Mapenterol	0.031	0.17	0.055
Ractopamine	0.36	1.45	0.41
Ritodrine	0.15	1.67	0.27
Salbutamol	0.13	3.45	0.44
Salmeterol	0.067	0.57	0.11
Sotalol	0.87	0.69	0.86
Terbutaline	0.46	Not calculable	2.54
Tulobuterol	0.041	0.15	0.09
Zilpaterol	0.40	0.35	0.23

Waters UPLC/Premier XE
UPLC
- Column: Acquity UPLC HSS T3 100 × 2.1, 1.8 µ
- Column temp.: 50 °C
- Flow: 450 µl/min
- Mobile phase A: 0.01% formic acid
- Mobile phase B: acetonitrile/0.01% formic acid = 95:5
- Gradient: 0.00–3 min 90% A, within 5 min to 70% A, remaining at 70% A for 1 min, within 4 min to 40% A, remaining at 40% A for 1 min, within 1 min to 90% A, 2 min at 90% A

Triple quad mass spectrometer
- Detection: MRM mode using ESI+ ionisation
- Capillary (kV) 3.00
- Extractor (V) 3.00
- RF Lens (V) 0.2
- Source Temperature (°C) 130
- Desolvation Temperature (°C) 450
- Cone Gas Flow (L/Hr) 77
- Desolvation Gas Flow (L/Hr) 802
- LM 1 Resolution 15.0
- HM 1 Resolution 13.0
- Ion Energy 1 0.5

Tab. 2-1 gives a comparison of the lowest concentration which can be confirmed if an API2000 system or a Quattro Premier XE systems is used. The resulting levels are compared with the CCα of the full validation on API4000.

Although the values for the Premier XE are slightly higher than for API 4000 the recommended concentrations are covered with this system too. The API 2000 does not meet the recommended concentrations for several compounds (e.g. clenbuterol, brombuterol, salbutamol).

Tab. 2-2 shows the results of a repeatability study using a tenfold injection of a processed urine sample fortified with 0.5 µg/kg. The repeatability of HP1100/API4000 and UPLC/Premier XE are comparable, whereas the values calculated for the HP1100/API2000 were clearly higher.

In summary the comparative study showed that confirmation method for β-agonists in urine can be extended to the UPLC/Premier XE system. In contrast to it the API2000 has some limitations. The validation data of this the sample preparation with API4000 detection cannot be transferred and would require a separate validation study, probably including a modified sample preparation procedure.

2.3
Validation of the method for 29 beta-agonists in retina by LC-MSMS

A method for the determination of β-agonists in retina was reworked and validated. The validation was performed on the basis of the matrix-comprehensive in-house validation procedure according to Commission Decision 2002/657/EC for retina of different species.

Tab. 2-2 Results of a repeatability study using a tenfold injection of a processed urine sample fortified with 0.5 µg/kg.

Analyte	API 4000® repeatability [%]	API 2000® repeatability [%]	Premier XE® repeatability [%]
Bamethan	6.96	16.00	8.71
Brombuterol	2.59	10.39	1.56
Bromchlorbuterol	1.99	11.05	2.24
Carbuterol	11.95	–	–
Cimaterol	3.43	11.76	3.16
Cimbuterol	4.03	9.07	3.99
Clenbuterol	3.49	11.55	3.19
Clencyclohexerol	3.03	10.82	3.55
Clenhexerol	2.66	12.76	3.10
Clenisopenterol	2.66	9.17	3.22
Clenpenterol	2.60	7.52	2.98
Clenproperol	2.41	5.97	2.12
Hydroxymethyl-clenb.	2.12	5.14	3.20
Fenoterol	5.78	15.34	5.18
Formoterol	4.02	12.43	4.11
Isoxsuprine	2.00	18.65	2.86
Labetalol	3.59	14.41	3.91
Mabuterol	2.66	7.57	2.54
Mapenterol	3.95	7.32	2.78
Ractopamine	4.54	18.67	4.00
Ritodrine	5.19	17.40	5.76
Salbutamol	5.58	15.95	4.59
Salmeterol	7.97	18.77	8.31
Sotalol	7.35	10.29	6.10
Terbutaline	8.48	–	9.91
Tulobuterol	2.39	8.98	2.93
Zilpaterol	5.23	13.37	6.88

The method is suitable for the confirmation and quantification of the same 26 β-agonists as described above in bovine and turkey retina. The experimental plan for the validation was established on the basis of the factors presented in *Tab. 2-3*.

Principle of the method:
Retina preparation
Retina is dissected from the eye and sub-samples (solutions of 1 ml in TRIS-buffer containing approx. 100 mg of retina) are prepared.

Sample pre-treatment
- Sub-samples of 100 mg are used
- 10 ml of TRIS-buffer are added
- Homogenisation
- Enzymatic digestion using protease at pH 8
- Solid-phase extraction using CleanScreenDau® cartridges
- LC-MS/MS measurement

HPLC parameters
- Column: Phenomenex LUNA C18, 150 × 2 mm, 3 µ
- Column temp.: 40 °C
- Flow: 300 µl/min
- Mobile phase A: 0.05 M ammonium formate in water, pH 4
- Mobile phase B: acetonitrile/0.05 M ammonium formate in water, pH 4 = 95:5
- Gradient: 0.00–3 min 90% A, within 7 min to 85% A, within 15 min to 60% A, within 3 min to 40% A, within 1 min to 90% A, 9 min at 90% A
- Injection volume: 20 µl
- Detection: MRM mode using ESI+ ionisation

UPLC can also be used with the following parameters:
- Column: Acquity UPLC HSS T3 100 × 2.1, 1.8 µ
- Column temp.: 50 °C
- Flow: 450 µl/min
- Mobile phase A: 0.01% formic acid
- Mobile phase B: acetonitrile/0.01% formic acid = 95:5
- Gradient: 0.00–3 min 90% A, within 5 min to 70% A, remaining at 70% A for 1 min, within 4 min to 40% A, remaining at 40% A for 1 min, within 1 min to 90% A, 2 min at 90% A
- Detection: MRM mode using ESI+ ionisation

The validation parameters are summarized in *Tab. 2-4*.

Tab. 2-3 Experimental plan for validation of the method for 29 beta-agonists in retina by LC-MSMS.

Leading factor:	species	bovine, turkey
Factors:	instrument	normal HPLC – fa-resolution HPLC
	storage conditions	frozen (–25 °C) – cooled (4 °C)
	duration of sample preparation	continuously – break before SPE
	storage of extracts	without – 2 d at 4 °C
	SPE	stainless steel cock – lead through
	solvent	HPLC-grade – UPLC-grade

Tab. 2-4 Summary of the validation parameters.

Analyte	CCα [ng/g]	CCβ [µg/kg]	Recovery [%]	RSD* [%]
Bamethan	0.84	1.42	114.6	20.8
Brombuterol	0.69	0.87	98.7	11.2
Bromchlorbuterol	0.64	0.75	97.6	8.5
Cimaterol	0.74	0.93	103.5	12.5
Cimbuterol	0.63	0.73	108.2	8.9
Clenbuterol	0.64	0.75	99.2	8.3
Clencyclohexerol	4.45	7.10	60.2	14.4
Clenhexerol	0.83	1.28	74.6	15.5
Clenisopenterol	0.75	1.00	90.0	13.3
Clenpenterol	0.66	0.81	91.2	9.4
Clenproperol	0.62	0.73	97.6	7.9
Hydroxymethyl-clenb.	0.89	1.57	77.9	20.5
Fenoterol	6.83	9.86	11.2	6.8
Formoterol	1.38	2.33	52.7	20.8
Isoxsuprine	0.803	1.203	89.7	17.1
Labetalol	3.712	6.071	86.1	21.0
Mabuterol	0.679	0.849	93.0	10.8
Mapenterol	0.626	0.731	95.2	7.7
Ractopamine	2.576	3.027	93.5	8.3
Ritodrine	1.239	3.666	55.9	22.5
Salbutamol	2.783	3.567	111.6	15.2
Salmeterol	2.558	3.061	102.2	9.5
Sotalol	0.751	0.944	86.5	10.6
Terbutaline	2.837	4.230	76.7	14.7
Tulobuterol	1.356	1.556	88.9	22.2
Zilpaterol	3.052	4.137	90.2	15.4

2.4 Optimisation and validation of method for 5 avermectins in aquaculture products

A method for the determination of 5 avermectins (abamectin, doramectin, emamectin, ivermectin and moxidectin) was newly developed and validated. The validation was performed on the basis of the matrix-comprehensive in-house validation procedure according to Commission Decision 2002/657/EC for salmon as well as for trout.

The validation was carried out for emamectin (MRL: 100 µg/kg) in a range of 25 µg/kg–200 µg/kg. The other four substances were validated in a concentration range of 1 µg/kg–15 µg/kg.

Principle of the method:
Sample pre-treatment
- 2 g of sample material are used
- Extraction with 10 ml of acetonitrile using a MefiFast homogeniser
- SPE on C18 cartridges
- Derivatisation with trifluoroacetic acid anhydride and N-methylimidazole
- Measurement by means of HPLC-FLU

HPLC parameters
- Column: two coupled Chromolith columns, 100 × 4.6 mm
- Column temp.: 40 °C
- Flow: 2000 µl/min
- Mobile phase A: acetonitrile/water/THF = 68/17/15
- Gradient: isokratic
- Injection volume: 20 µl
- Detection: FLU:(EX: 365 nm, EM: 455 nm)

The experimental plan for the validation was established on the basis of the factors presented in Tab. 2-5. The summary of the validation parameters for the validation method for 5 avermectins in aquaculture products is presented in Tab. 2-6.

Tab. 2-5 Factors for the experimental plan for the validation method for 5 avermectins in aquaculture products.

Leading factor:	species	trout, salmon
Factors:	operator	Maidhof – Matthes
	instrument	FLU – FLU/ADC
	storage conditions	frozen – 4 °C
	cartridge lot	old – new
	duration of sample preparation	without break – 1 day break before SPE
	storage of injection solution	without – 2 days at 4 °C

Tab. 2-6 Summary of the validation parameters for the validation method for 5 avermectins in aquaculture products.

Analyte	CCα [ng/g]	CCβ [µg/kg]	Recovery [%]	RSD [%]
Abamectin	1.415	1.813	101.2	13.2
Doramectin	1.424	1.836	100.7	13.9
Emamectin	127.355	153.733	90.9	9.4
Ivermectin	1.364	1.708	99.3	12.5
Moxidectin	1.741	2.378	108.4	19.3

2.5 Long term stability studies for all substance groups

2.5.1 Anticoccidials

Long term stability study in lyophilised egg was performed with following analytes: narasin, dinitrocarbanilide (marker for nicarbazin) and monensin. The material was produced in 2003 and stored for five years at –25 °C and –80 °C as reference material. *Fig. 2-5* shows the results for the five years storage. In contrast to monensin and dinitrocarbanilide narasin shows a decomposition after storage of five years, even at a storage temperature of –80 °C.

2.5.2 Avermectines

Long term stability study in lyophilised milk was performed with following analytes: ivermectin, moxidectin, doramectin and eprinomectin. For that purpose the incurred material was

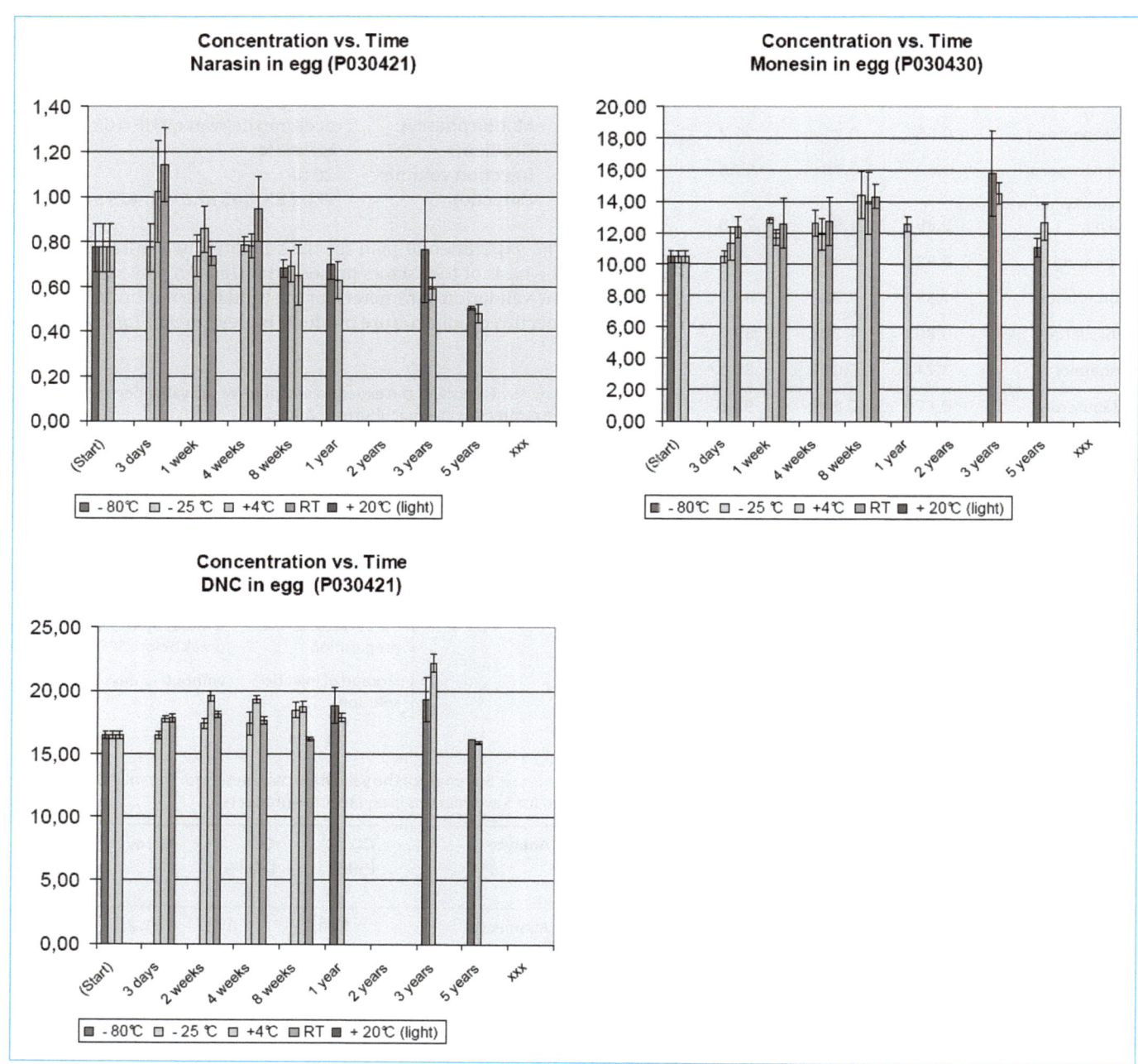

Fig. 2-5 Results for the five years storage of the anticoccidials Narasin, Monesin and DNC.

Tab. 2-7 Stability of avermectines (Ivermectin, Moxidectin, Doramectin, Eprinomectin) during three years storage.

Sample	Analyte	Target value 2005 [µg/kg]	Target value 2008 [µg/kg]
P050140	Ivermectin	1,000	0.843
	Moxidectin	27.88	26.10
P050141	Doramectin	2.69	2.76
	Moxidectin	14.58	14.54
P050144	Eprinomectin	1.05	1.17
	Moxidectin	32.58	35.73

stored at −20 °C for three years. In 2005 the material was used for a proficiency test with 37 participants. 2008 the samples were re-evaluated. The comparison of the results of 2005 and 2008 shows (Tab. 2-7) that the examined analytes are stable at least for three years if the material is stored at −25 °C.

2.5.3 Benzimidazoles

Stability studies in lyophilised milk were performed with the following analytes:

- Albendazole (ALBZ) and its metabolites albendazole sulfoxide (ALBZSO), albendazole sulphone (ALBZSO2) and albendazole 2-aminosulphone (ALBZ-NH2SO2)
- Fenbendazole (FEBZ) and its metabolites oxfendazole (OFEB) and oxfendazole sulphone (O2FEB)
- Triclabendazole (TCBZ) and its metabolites triclabendazole sulfoxide (TCBZSO), triclabendazole sulphone (TCBZSO2) and ketotriclabendazole (K-TCBZ)
- Levamisole (LEV)

For short-term stability (4 weeks) the samples were stored in brown glass vials with screw caps and septum at −80 °C (reference temperature), −25 °C, +4 °C and +20 °C (dark). For long-term stability for up to two years the samples were stored at −25 °C and +4 °C. In general the samples are stable for at least four weeks at all chosen storage conditions. Details on the realisation of the stability studies and their results will be documented on information sheets and published in FIS-VL as well as in the report on results of PT "Anthelmintics in Cow's milk". The results of the long-term stability study are published in FIS-VL.

2.5.4 Nitroimidazoles

Long-term/short-term stability studies with nitroimidazoles and their hydroxy-metabolites were carried out in lyophilised turkey muscle, in lyophilised pig plasma and in lyophilised whole egg.

a) in lyophilised pig plasma
A lyophilised mixture of different incurred plasma samples containing dimetridazole, metronidazole, ipronidazole and their hydroxy-metabolites was stored at different temperatures (−25 °C, +4 °C, +25 °C, isochronous approach with −80 °C as reference temperature) for 1 year. There was no significant degradation within this period.

b) in lyophilised turkey muscle
Different incurred muscle samples were mixed, lyophilised and stored for five years in brown glass vials with screw caps. Storage temperature: −25 °C.

Three different samples containing ipronidazole, ronidazole and their hydroxy-metabolites as well as ipronidazole, dimetridazole and their hydroxy-metabolites were tested. The analytes proved to be stable when stored at −25 °C for at least five years.

c) in lyophilised whole egg
Different incurred whole egg samples were mixed, lyophilised and stored at different temperatures (−25 °C, +4 °C, +25 °C, isochronous approach with −80 °C as reference temperature) for one year in brown glass vials with screw caps. There was no significant degradation within this period.

In addition stability studies of lyophilised porc muscle material were performed within the framework of the production of a CRM for nitroimidazoles (C3); the stability of the analytes in fresh chicken muscle was investigated during the animal study as described above.

2.5.5 NSAIDs

Stability studies were performed with the following analytes (basic NSAIDs):

marker metabolite of metamizole – 4-methylaminoantipyrine (MAA),
further metabolites: antipyrine (A); 4-aminoantipyrene (AA);
N-acetylaminoantipyrene (AAA); 4-hydroxyantipyrene (4OH-A);
4-formylaminoantipyrene (FAA); dimethylaminoantipyrene (DMAA),
as well as isopropylaminoantipyrene (IPAA); isoprppylantipyrine (PPHZ) and aminopropylone (APP),
including the internal deuterated standards MAA-d3; AA-d3; A-d3; IPAA-d3,
as well as DMAA-13C2.

The standard solutions were stored for up to four weeks (short-term stability) in brown glass vials with screw caps and septum at −80 °C (reference temperature), −20 °C, +4 °C, +20 °C (dark) and +20 °C (daylight) in different solutions. The example (Fig. 2-6) shows a degradation of the marker metabolite MAA in acetonitrile already at −20 °C and +4 °C of up to 35% within 4 weeks.

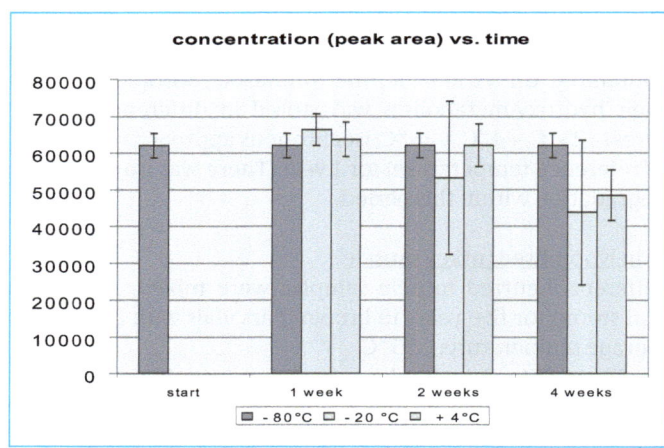

Fig. 2-6 The degradation of the marker metabolite MAA in acetonitrile already at −20 °C and +4 °C of up to 35% within 4 weeks.

Details on the realisation of the stability studies was repeated and is documented on information sheets and in FIS-VL.

Further stability studies were performed with the following analyte/matrix combinations:

- phenylbutazone (PBZ) in bovine muscle from 2006 (incurred material – lyophilised and fresh – stored at −20 °C)
- Diclofenac (DC) and meloxicam (MLX) in bovine muscle from 2004 (incurred fresh material – stored at −20 °C)

There was no significant degradation within this period. The studies are being continued.

Further quality control materials were produced from incurred milk with the marker residue MAA and further metabolites of metamizole (4-aminoantipyrene (AA); 4-formylaminoantipyrene (FAA) and 4-hydroxyantipyrene (4OH-A)). This material will be used for internal quality control charts:

a) P080301 (fresh and lyophilised): with about 30 µg/kg MAA; 20 µg/kg FAA and 10 µg/kg AA

b) P080299 (fresh): with about 500 µg/kg MAA; 120 µg/kg FAA; 60 µg/kg AA and 10 µg/kg 4-OH-A.

These materials will be checked regularly and were available for quality control purposes.

2.6
Research and identification of new or unknown compounds

In 2008 a HPLC-QTOF system was purchased and successfully put into operation. The investigation of samples for new substances was started; these samples had yielded positive screening results in the MRM-mode, which could not be confirmed. Also in 2008 some new substances were tested as analytes or internal standards.

2.6.1 Benzimidazoles

The synthesis of some new deuterated standards was initialized and introduced into the method: Febendazole-d3, oxfendazole-d3, oxfendazole sulphone-d3, mebendazole-d3, hydroxymebendazole-d3, oxibendazole-d7, amino oxibendazole-d7, flubendazole–d3.

2.6.2 Coccidiostats

Robenidine-d7, decoquinat-d5.

2.6.3 NSAIDs

To allow a better identification of NSAIDs, new deuterated standards (firocoxib-d6; carprofen-d3; 4-aminoantipyrine-d3) as well as tolfenamic acid-13C6 and one of the metabolites of metamizole (4-hydroxyantipyrene) were bought.

3 Quality assurance and quality control including the development of incurred test material and the organisation of a proficiency test[1]

3.1 Maintenance of equipment, documentation, audits, management

The adaptation of the quality control system is conducted continuously. SOPs are revised, e.g. on the "treatment of samples", "archiving of documents", "pipettes", "establishment of test reports" and "computer-aided systems". Staff was trained. The maintenance of instruments is performed continuously. Preparations were made for the re-accreditation in 2009.

To prove our competence we participated in the following proficiency tests: ***Participation in proficiency tests (in addition to work programme 2008)***
- The CRL participated in the proficiency test on anthelmintics (benzimidazoles and levamisole) in milk 'ANTH_04/08' – successful,
- CRL interlaboratory study on avermectins in milk – successful.

The CRL is also participated in proficiency tests from other PT-providers. The following proficiency tests demonstrate the competence of the entire lab:
- Proficiency test Progetto Trieste; β-agonists in urine; 03.11.08 – successful,
- Certification study IRMM on nitroimidazoles in muscle; September 2008 – successful.

3.2 Proficiency test on benzimidazoles in milk: characterisation of the material, packaging, evaluation

Official residue control laboratories have to prove their competence by regularly participating in proficiency tests organised or recognised by NRLs or CRLs. These proficiency tests provide the participating laboratories with the opportunity to check their routine test methods and thus contribute to an objective evaluation of the performance of these laboratories.

The interlaboratory study on anthelmintics in milk was prepared and organised during this reference period. The test material consisted of five milk samples (lyophilised samples) containing incurred residues of albendazole (ALBZ), fenbendazole (FEBZ), triclabendazole (TCBZ), levamisole (LEV) and their metabolites as well as of one blank sample. All samples were produced by mixing incurred with blank material. The animals were kept at the holding for test animals of the *Zentrum für experimentelle Tierhaltung* (centre for experimental animal husbandry) of the Federal Institute for Risk Assessment (BfR) and were treated with commercially available preparations as described in the report. The tests on homogeneity and stability were performed according to international standards.

On 01 April 2008 the sample material was shipped to 28 laboratories (19 National Reference Laboratories (NRLs), 3 German Routine Field Laboratories (RFLs) and 6 official laboratories from Third Countries. In total 27 laboratories submitted results (19 labs from MS (NRL), 2 German RFLs and 6 official laboratories from Third Countries – Serbia, Russia, Norway, Thailand and Chile (3×). 7 MS did not answer (DK, IT and MT) or cancelled their participation (FI, RO, SE and UK). The deadline for the submission of the results was 15 May 2008.

Thirteen (10 NRLs, one official laboratory from Third Countries (Russia) and two German RFLs) of the 23 laboratories having performed a confirmatory analysis achieved satisfying results. Their analytical spectrum covered all the substances present in the samples; furthermore these laboratories generally performed a good quantification of all analytes. Eight of them suffered comparatively small deductions for deviations from the median of all laboratories (deviation greater than the simple HORWITZ standard deviation for the MRL substances

---
[1] Annex V, chapter 2, section 1 (a, b, c, g)

albendazole and fenbendazole – |z-score| > 1, as well as for the non-authorised substance triclabendazole – |z_u-scores| > 2).

Ten laboratories (seven NRLs and three official laboratory from Third Countries) having performed a confirmatory analysis submitted unsatisfactory results. These laboratories had failed to include several substances, or, respectively, performed an insufficient quantification of the MRL substances albendazole and fenbendazole and of the non-authorised substances triclabendazole and levamisole.

Regarding the four laboratories (two NRLs, two TCs) which exclusively applied screening methods, it can be stated that the HPLC-DAD and -FLD methods they used only fulfil the requirements for certain substances. To be used for confirmatory purposes these methods need to be revised and validated; moreover further analytes need to be covered, including the marker residues for albendazole, fenbendazole and triclabendazole.

The evaluation of this proficiency test shows that HPLC-MS/MS methods are particularly suited for the analysis of anthelmintics. Three laboratories which successfully carried out the analysis by means of HPLC-DAD and HPLC-FLD methods, proved that these methods can also still be applied for certain anthelmintic substances.

The participants were informed on their results by means of short preliminary reports, which they were asked to confirm, and a final report on results.

3.3
Cooperation with IRMM for the production of CRM for nitroimidazoles

In 2007 the IRMM started a characterization study of the candidate ERM. The CRL Berlin was one of the participating laboratories. The results have meanwhile been published (ERM-BB124 certification report). The analyte concentrations detected in the samples were in good agreement with the certified values of the material.

As a prerequisite for the release of the ERM the shelf life of the material has to be estimated on the basis of a long-term stability study. The CRL Berlin performed these stability studies, the results were in good agreement with earlier results of homogeneity and stability studies. A sufficient stability of the material could be estimated by the IRMM, and the certified material was released.

3.4
Production of incurred sample material

3.4.1 Avermectins in aquaculture
The material from an animal study (two avermectins in trout) was tested. It will be stored for the production of in-house reference material.

3.4.2 Nitroimidazoles in hens

Hens were treated with different nitroimidazoles (ronidazole, metronidazole, tinidazole, carnidazole). Muscle, liver and plasma/serum samples were collected and analysed.

The amount of incurred matrix material obtained from the animals of the study was not sufficient (with respect to the amount of material and the amount of detected residues) for the production of an in-house reference material. Anyhow the material is at least suitable for qualitative analysis checks and will be stored for additional tests.

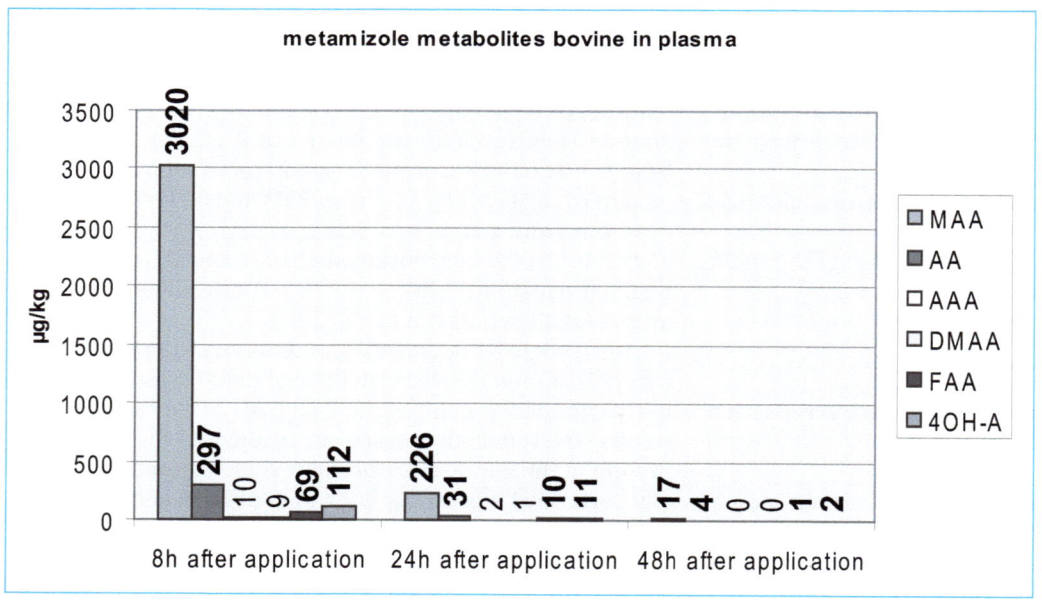

Fig. 3-1 Decrease of the amount of the marker metabolite (MAA) from about 3000 µg/kg (8 hours) to about 20 µg/kg within 48 hours after application in plasma.

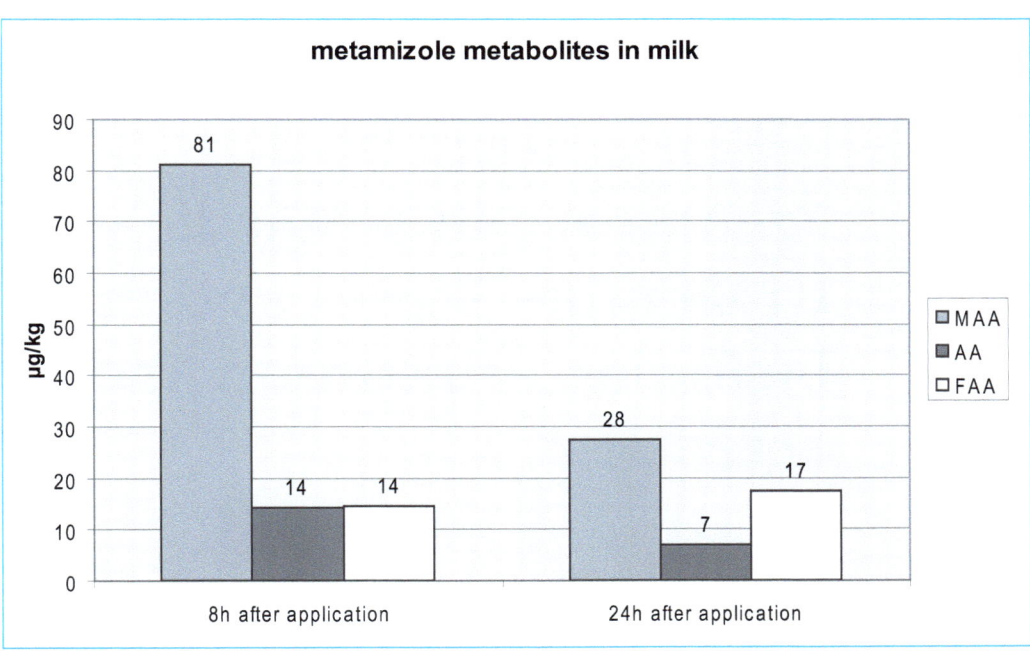

Fig. 3-2 Decrease of the amount of 4-methylaminoantipyrine (MAA) in milk below the MRL of 50 µg within 24 hours (further details in the text).

3.4.3 Beta-agonists in cattle (hair and urine)

Material was produced from an animal study (six β-agonists in bovine urine and hair). It is under ongoing examination. After finishing the tests it will be stored for the production of in-house reference material. In order to produce homogeneous hair material a special stainless steel ball mill was purchased.

3.4.4 NSAIDs (metamizole) in milk and plasma (in addition to work plan)

The material from an animal study (dairy cow – treated with metamizole) was examined and tested for metabolites of metamizole.

The marker metabolite 4-methylaminoantipyrine (MAA) as well as the further metabolites 4-aminoantipyrene (AA); 4-hydroxyantipyrene (4OH-A); 4-formylaminoantipyrene (FAA) as well as traces of dimethylaminoantipyrene (DMAA) and N-acetylaminoantipyrene (AAA) could be confirmed in plasma with the help of the internal standards MAA-d3; AA-d3; A-d3; IPAA-d3 and DMAA-13C2. The amount of the marker metabolite (MAA) decreased from about 3000 µg/kg (8 hours) to about 20 µg/kg within 48 hours after application in plasma (*Fig. 3-1*). The marker metabolite 4-methylaminoantipyrine (MAA) as well as the further metabolites 4-aminoantipyrene (AA) and 4-formylaminoantipyrene (FAA) could be confirmed in milk.

The amount of MAA decreases below the MRL of 50 µg within 24 hours (*Fig. 3-2*). The further metabolites FAA and AA should be considered for the control of compliance.

The milk samples were lyophilised and used for further methodical tests and for the production of in-house reference material. The material will be used for internal quality assurance purposes (method validation and control charts) and is available for other NRLs or RFLs.

4 Technical and scientific support to Member States and the Commission including arbitration and training activities[1]

4.1
Technical, scientific support and training

The CRL Berlin continued to provide training courses to scientists from EU Member States and Germany:

27.–29.02.08	Nitroimidazoles in egg, 2 participants from the NRL in Bratislava, Slovakia
21.–25.04.08	NSAIDs in milk and plasma, 1 participant from the Veterinary Faculty of the University of Ljubljana, Slovenia
18.11.08	Benzimidazoles in muscle and liver; 1 participant from the RFL in Rostock, Germany
01.–05.12.08	NSAIDs in muscle, liver and kidney; avermectins in liver, 1 participant from the NRL in Nicosia, Cyprus
08.–09.12.08	NSAIDs in muscle, liver and kidney; 2 participants from the NRL in Bratislava, Slovakia

Furthermore extensive telephone and e-mail support was provided to EC and Third Country laboratories. Visits of different scientists take place introducing them to the European reference laboratory system and/or showing them through the laboratory (Tab. 4-1).

Maintenance and improvement of the German *Fachinformationssystem Vebraucherschutz und Lebensmittelsicherheit*, FIS-VL (Information System Consumer Protection and Food Safety), which is based on the European CIRCA platform, were ongoing.

The system offers an up-to-date online access for official residue laboratories as well as their competent authorities. The information is provided in English and includes all aspects of residue control, e.g. programmes and reports, workshops, interlaboratory studies, publications, legal texts, test methods, reference materials, standard substances, studies on stability etc.

To maintain a high level of protection of the information provided, all members are checked once a year for access validity.

4.2
Follow-up of proficiency test

In response to the preliminary reports and the presentation during the workshop, the laboratories furnished additional information on method details and analytical results.

The final report on results was prepared and shipped. The participants therewith received a questionnaire offering further follow-up measures (e.g. provision of test methods, standards and defined sample material, support through training measures and workshops etc.).

4.3
Provision of standard substances, reference materials and methods, incl. procuring, storage, administration, documentation, shipment etc.

4.3.1 Standard Substances[2]

In accordance with the responsibilities laid down in Council Directive 96/23/EC of 29 April 1996, the CRL/NRL Berlin provided 948 units of reference standards (825 thereof in its responsibility as CRL) to the NRLs in the EU Member States, to Third Countries as well as to official residue control laboratories in Germany during this reference period. Standard substances of a total value of 71,828 € for the CRL/NRL (34,736 € thereof for CRL tasks) were procured. They had to be financed from the BVL budget.

---

[1] Annex V, chapter 2, section 1 (d, f, h, l)

[2] Annex V, chapter 2, section 1 (a, f)

Tab. 4-1 Visits of different scientists introducing them to the European reference laboratory system and/or showing them through the laboratory.

Date	Participants	Institute and Country	Purpose of visit
30.06.08	Dr. C. Cerdchu +1	National Institute of Metrology (Thailand)	visit of laboratory
13.11.08	Frau Dr. Weiß + staff + students	Humboldt-Universität zu Berlin, Landwirtschaftlich-gärtnerische Fakultät, Gemeinschaftslabor Analytik	visit of the laboratory in the framework of a university seminar

Tab. 4-2 Incurred in-house reference materials provided to various recipients in 2008.

Sample material	Quantity	Substance (group)	Recipient	Date
Bovine, milk (lyo) AVER_07/05	6 × 5 g	Avermectins	Croatian Veterinary Institute	2008-01-07
Egg (lyo) NIIM_09/07	4 × 2.4 g	Nitroimidazoles	State Veterinary and Food Institute, Bratislava, Slovak Republic	2008-01-22
Shrimps (lyo) / Muscle (fresh)	1 × 4.3 g / 2 × 30 g	CAP / Tetracyclines	Institut für Hygiene und Umwelt, Hamburg, Germany	2008-04-08
Pig, plasma (lyo)	2 × 1.2 g	Nitroimidazoles	State Laboratory, Dublin, Ireland	2008-04-14
Pig, plasma (lyo)	2 × 1.2 g	Nitroimidazoles	Laboratory Central Agricultural Office / Food and Feed Safety Directorate / Budapest, Hungary	2008-06-23
Egg (lyo) NIIM_09/07	4 × 2.4 g	Nitroimidazoles	Laboratory Central Agricultural Office Food and Feed Safety Directorate Budapest, Hungary	2008-06-23
Pig, plasma (lyo)	2 × 1.2 g	Nitroimidazoles	Norwegian School of Veterinary Science; Oslo, Norway	2008-06-24
Egg (lyo)	4 × 2.6 g	Nitrofuranes	Norwegian School of Veterinary Science; Oslo, Norway	2008-06-24
Milk (lyo)	1 × 6.4 g; 1 × 7.05 g (50 ml)	NSAIDs (Metamizole)	Bayerisches Gesundheitsamt, Oberschleißheim (BY), Germany	2008-10-20
Bovine, plasma (NSAI_06/02)/ Bovine, muscle/ milk (lyo)	3 × 4.25 g / 2 × 5 g / 6 × 5 g	NSAIDs	State Laboratory, Dublin, Ireland	2008-11-21
Shrimps (lyo) / Bovine, urine (fresh) / milk (lyo)	3 × 4.3 g / 2 × 50 ml / 8 × 6.0 g	CAP / β-Agonists / Avermectins	State General Laboratory, Nicosia, Cyprus	2008-12-05
Bovine, plasma (NSAI_06/02)	3 × 4.25 g	NSAIDs	State Veterinary and Food Institute, Bratislava, Slovak Republic	2008-12-09

4.3.2 Shipment of in-house reference materials[3]

Incurred in-house reference materials were provided to various recipients (*Tab. 4-2*). In total more than 53 samples of in-house reference material with incurred residues of avermectins, β-agonists, nitroimidazoles and NSAIDs were sent to laboratories in the Slovak Republic, Ireland, Hungary, Cyprus, Croatia, Norway and Germany (Hamburg and Oberschleißheim).

4.3.3 Shipment of test methods[4]

In total 33 methods for the analysis of nitroimidazoles, β-agonists, avermectins, benzimidazoles, NSAIDs and coccidiostats were sent to 16 laboratories in Spain, Poland, UK, France, Cyprus, Slovak Republic, Canada, Russia and Germany (Arnsberg, Chemnitz, Frankfurt, Oberschleißheim and Hannover) (*Tab. 4-3*). Moreover, the methods available at the CRL can be found in the FIS-VL and can be downloaded anytime.

---

[3] Annex V, chapter 2, section 1 (a, b)

[4] Annex V, chapter 2, section 1 (a, b)

Tab. 4-3 List of methods for the analysis of nitroimidazoles, ß-agonists, avermectins, benzimidazoles, NSAIDs and coccidiostats, which were sent to 16 laboratories in 2008.

0.	Method code	Additional information	Analyte/matrix	Recipient	Date
1.	BETA_013, BETA_014	Method description	Urine / Liver	Public Health Laboratory, Zamora, ES	2008-01-07
2.	NSAI_007	Method description	Milk	National Veterinary Research Institute, Pulawy, PL	2008-01-10
3.	AVER_001 AVER_002 AVER_003	Method description Short description	Milk; Muscle	Técnico Superior de Laboratorio, Lugo, ES	2008-01-22
4.	BETA_013, BETA_014	Method description	Urine / Liver	Central Meat Control Laboratory, Celbridge, Co. Kildare, UK	2008-01-23
5.	basic NSAIDs	Short description	Milk	RFL Arnsberg, NRW, DE	2008-02-14
6.	BENZ_003	Short description	Milk	RFL Chemnitz, SN, DE	2008-03-05
7.	BENZ_003	Short description	Milk	Agence Francaise de Sécurite Sanitaire des Aliments (AFSSA), Fougères, FR	2008-03-20
8.	AVER_001 AVER_003 BENZ_003	Method description Short description	Milk; Muscle	RFL Frankfurt, BB, DE	2008-03-21
9.	COCC_002 COCC_004	Method description	Egg, Muscle and liver	RFL Oberschleißheim, BY, DE	2008-04-08
10.	NIIM_009	Method description Short description	Muscle, Plasma	Canadian Food Inspection Agency, Canada	2008-04-10
11.	AVER_001 AVER_002 AVER_003	Method description Short description	Milk; Muscle, Liver	The All-Russia State Centre for Quality and Standardization of Veterinary Drugs and Feed (VGNKI), Moscow, Russia	2008-04-21
12.	NSAI_004	Method description (Poster)	Muscle, Liver, Kidney	State Veterinary and Food Institute Bratislava; SK	2008-10-23
13.	Avermectins	Method description (Literature)	Milk and liver	RFL, Oberschleißheim, BY, DE	2008-11-25
14.	Avermectins	Method description (Literature)	Milk and liver	RFL, Hannover, NI, DE	2008-11-25
15.	NSAID_004; AVER_001; AVER_003; AVER_003	Method description	NSAIDs in muscle, liver and kidney; Avermectins in milk and liver	State General Laboratory; Nicosia, CY	2008-12-04
16.	NSAID_004; MAA_002	Method description	NSAIDs in muscle, liver and kidney; MAA in plasma and tissue	StateVeterinary and Food Institute; Bratislava, SK	2008-12-09

4.4 Analysis of official samples

In total 19 samples were requested in 2008: (a) 7 samples for β-agonists in turkey liver, (b) 10 samples for β-agonists in urine liver, (c) 2 samples for β-agonists in bovine retina. The analyses were requested by NRLs of Ireland and Belgium for confirmatory purposes. No counter analyses for arbitration were requested in 2008.

4.5 Visit to NRLs

In June 2008 a three-day supporting visit to the NRL in Budapest/Hungary, took place. The NRL was interested in a co-operation, especially regarding the implementation/enhancement of methods for nitroimidazoles, avermectins, benzimidazoles and β-agonists, measurement uncertainty, stability testing etc., and in information on method validation. Methods for the determination of nitroimidazoles in eggs and a multi-method for β-agonists in urine were demonstrated. A report was issued and sent to the Commission.

4.6 Organisation and realisation of a Workshop: measurement uncertainty, analytical news and problems

4.6.1 Objective

The workshop of the CRL Berlin was again an opportunity to forward the latest information on legal developments and on the residue analysis of benzimidazoles and nitroimidazoles to the appropriate addressees, namely the National Reference Laboratories, for further dissemination.

The draft guideline on the assessment of positive results of substances with sum-MRL was presented and discussed as well as the validation of screening methods. Furthermore new developments in the field of avermectins and benzimidazoles and their detection by LC-MSMS as well as in the field of method-automisation were discussed.

4.6.2 Course of the Workshop

The programme of the Workshop, the main topics of the presentations and the list of participants as well as some useful supplementary information were compiled in the Workshop manual, which was handed out to all participants at the beginning of the Workshop. The main topics covered were:
1. Overview of the activities of the CRL Berlin in 2007 and the activities planned for 2008, taking into account the results of the questionnaire of Workshop 04/07,
2. Developments in Community residue control legislation,
3. Evaluation of NRCPs of the MS,
4. Validation of screening methods,
5. Sum-MRL,
6. List of recommended concentrations,
7. Animal study on nitroimidazoles in hens,
8. Results of proficiency test NIIM_06/07 and consequences as regards the follow-up procedure prescribed by COM,
9. Avermectins – use, analytical aspects,
10. Stability testing at the CRL Berlin,
11. Practical exercise: Benzimidazoles in tissue (participation on voluntary basis).

4.6.3 Evaluation

As in previous years the participants emphasised the importance of these workshops for the exchange of information and the possibility to get into contact with colleagues from other NRLs, especially during breaks and during practical work.

Many participants found that the workshop provided new information to them (56%), which they can use, or partly use, in their laboratories (84%).

The participation of the EC representative was highly acknowledged. On the one hand, it underlines the importance the Commission attributes to these workshops, on the other hand, it allows the discussion of legal questions and of questions with regard to the interpretation of certain rules. A workshop report was submitted to the Commission.

4.7 Publications, reports and contributions

Bohm, D., Hamann, F., Stoyke, M., Hackenberg, R. and Stachel, C. (2008a) Preparation and Characterisation of In-house Reference Material for Antibiotics in Bovine Milk. Proceedings Volume 3, Euroresidue VI – Conference on Residues of Veterinary Drugs in Food; Egmond aan Zee, The Netherlands, 19 to 21 May 2008; page 1187–1191.

Bohm, D., Xia, X., Stoyke, M., Stachel, C. and Gowik, P. (2008b) Multi-Method for the Determination of Antibiotics of Different Substance Groups in Milk and Validation in Accordance with CD 2002/657/EC. Proceedings Volume 3, Euroresidue VI – Conference on Residues of Veterinary Drugs in Food; Egmond aan Zee, The Netherlands, 19 to 21 May 2008; page 1193–1199.

Gowik, P. (2008) The State of and Update on Commission Decision 2002/657/EC. Proceedings Volume 1, Euroresidue VI – Conference on Residues of Veterinary Drugs in Food; Egmond aan Zee, The Netherlands, 19 to 21 May 2008; page 131–136.

Gowik, P., Polzer, J. and Uhlig, S. (2008) Determination of MU in Residue Analysis by Means of a Statistical Factorial Design. Proceedings Volume 3, Euroresidue VI – Conference on Residues of Veterinary Drugs in Food; Egmond aan Zee, The Netherlands, 19 to 21 May 2008; page 1205–1209.

Hackenberg, R., Bohm, D., Hamann, F., Stachel, C. and Gowik, P. (2008) Evaluation of a Proficiency Test on the Determination of Tetracyclines and Quinolones in Milk. Proceedings Volume 3, Euroresidue VI – Conference on Residues of Veterinary Drugs in Food; Egmond aan Zee, The Netherlands, 19 to 21 May 2008; page 1201–1204.

Polzer, J., Hamann, F., Neumärker, A. and Gowik, P. (2008) Control of Nitroimidazole Residues in Food of Animal Origin: Overview of Recent Results on Suitable Matrices, Analyte Stability and Metabolisation. Proceedings Volume 1, Euroresidue VI – Conference on Residues of Veterinary Drugs in Food; Egmond aan Zee, The Netherlands, 19 to 21 May 2008; page 47–52.

Polzer, J., Henrion, A., Garrido, S., Stoyke, M. and Gowik, P. (2008) Interlaboratory study chloramphenicol in milk: results of routine field laboratories and National Metrology Institutes. Proceedings Volume 1, Euroresidue VI – Conference on Residues of Veterinary Drugs in Food; Egmond aan Zee, The Netherlands, 19 to 21 May 2008; page 1217.

Radeck, W. and Gowik, P. (2008) Validation of a Multi-residue Method for the Confirmation and Quantification of Anthelmintics in Milk. Proceedings Volume 3, Euroresidue VI – Conference on Residues of Veterinary Drugs in Food; Egmond aan Zee, The Netherlands, 19 to 21 May 2008; page 1181–1186.

Report on laboratories' performances within the FVO report on the mission to Spain. (not yet published)

Report on activities of the CRL Berlin in 2007. Annual report to the European Commission, DG SANCO. March 2008. http://europa.eu.int/comm/food/fs/sfp/crl_residues_en.html.

Schmidt, K. S., Stachel, C. and Gowik, P. (2008) Validation and Multivariate Effect Analysis of an LC-MS/MS Method for the Determination of Steroids in Bovine Muscle. Proceedings Volume 1, Euroresidue VI – Conference on Residues of Veterinary Drugs in Food; Egmond aan Zee, The Netherlands, 19 to 21 May 2008; page 145–150.

Stoyke, M., Polzer, J., Hamann, F., Neumärker, A., Garrido, S. and Gowik, P. (2007a) Nitroimadazoles in Egg (Lyophilised Samples) – Interlaboratory Study NIIM_09/07. Report on Results, January 2008, page 1–73.

Stoyke, M., J. Polzer, J., Hamann, F., Neumärker, A., Garrido, S. and Gowik, P. (2007b) Nitroimidazole im Vollei (Lyophilisat) – Laborvergleichsstudie NIIM_09/07. Ergebnis-bericht, Januar 2008, Seite 1–73.

Stoyke, M. and Gowik, P. (2008a) Ten Years of Interlaboratory Studies in the Field of Analysis of not permitted and authorized Veterinary Drugs. Eurachem – 6th Workshop Proficiency Testing in Anal. Chemistry, Microbiol. and Lab. Medicine, Rome, Italy, 05 to 07 October 2008.

Stoyke, M., Radeck, W., Hamann, F. and Gowik, P. (2008b) Avermectine in Kuhmilch (Lyophilisat) – Laborvergleich 2008. Ergebnisbericht, November 2008, Seite 1–41.

Stoyke, M.; W. Radeck; F. Hamann and P. Gowik (2008c): "Anthelmintics in Cow's Milk (Lyophilised Samples) – Interlaboratory Study ANTH_04/08", Report on Results, December 2008, page 1–84.

Stoyke, M.; W. Radeck; F. Hamann and P. Gowik (2008d): „Anthelmintika in Kuhmilch (Lyophilisat) – Laborvergleichsstudie ANTH_04/08", Ergebnisbericht, Dezember 2008, Seite 1–84.

Stoyke, M., Radeck, W., Hamann, F. and Gowik, P. (2008e) Interlaboratory study – Coccidiostats in Egg. Proceedings Volume 3, Euroresidue VI – Conference on Residues of Veterinary Drugs in Food; Egmond aan Zee, The Netherlands, 19 to 21 May 2008; page 1163–1167.

Stoyke, M., Polzer, J., Hamann, F., Garrido, S. and Gowik, P. (2008f) Interlaboratory study – Nitroimidazoles in Egg. Proceedings Volume 3, Euroresidue VI – Conference on Residues of Veterinary Drugs in Food; Egmond aan Zee, The Netherlands, 19 to 21 May 2008; page 1175–1179.

Stoyke, M., Polzer, J., Radeck, W., Hamann, F. and Gowik, P. (2008g) Potential and Limits of the Statistical Evaluation of Proficiency Tests. Proceedings Volume 3, Euroresidue VI – Conference on Residues of Veterinary Drugs in Food; Egmond aan Zee, The Netherlands, 19 to 21 May 2008; page 1169–1173.

Workshop Manual: "On Analytical and Statistical Issues", CRL Workshop Berlin, 03 to 06 June 2008.

Working Plan of the CRL Berlin for Residues for 2009. Annual report to the European Commission, DG SANCO. August 2007. http://europa.eu.int/comm/food/fs/sfp/crl_residues_en.html

4.8
Presentations

Gowik, P. (2008a) Introduction and general topics – Overview of technical and organisational work of the CRL in 2007. CRL-Workshop 2008, Berlin, 03 to 06 June 2008.

Gowik, P. (2008b) State of and Update on Commission Decision 2002/657/EC – presentation held at EuroResidue VI. CRL-Workshop 2008, Berlin, 03 to 06 June 2008.

Gowik, P. (2008c) News on Sum-MRL. CRL-Workshop 2008, Berlin, 03 to 06 June 2008.

Gowik, P. (2008d) Neues aus der Kommission und Bericht vom CRL-Workshop in Berlin. NRL Fachtagung 2008, Berlin, 17 to 18 June 2008.

Gowik, P. (2008e) Validierung von Screeningmethoden. NRL Fachtagung 2008, Berlin, 17 to 18 June 2008.

Polzer, J. (2008a) Results of a CCQM Pilot Study in Milk. CRL-Workshop 2008, Berlin, 03 to 06 June 2008.

Polzer, J. (2008b) News on Nitroimidazoles. CRL-Workshop 2008, Berlin, 3 to 6 June 2008

Polzer, J. (2008c) Control of Nitroimidazole Residues in Food of Animal Origin: Overview of Recent Results on Suitable Matrices, Analyte Stability and Metabolisation. Euroresidue VI – Conference on Residues of Veterinary Drugs in Food; Egmond aan Zee, The Netherlands, 19 May 2008.

Polzer, J. (2008d) Ergebnisse der CCQM Pilotstudie – CAP in Milch. NRL Fachtagung 2008, Berlin, 17 to 18 June 2008.

Polzer, J. (2008e) Neues zum Thema Nitroimidazole. NRL Fachtagung 2008, Berlin, 17 to 18 June 2008.

Radeck, W. (2008a) Evaluation of NRCP – Group A5, B2a and B2b substances. CRL-Workshop 2008, Berlin, 03 to 06 June 2008.

Radeck, W. (2008b) Avermectins in Fish – Method and Additional Information. CRL-Workshop 2008, Berlin, 03 to 06 June 2008.

Radeck, W. (2008c) Avermectine in Fisch. NRL Fachtagung 2008, Berlin, 17/18 June 2008.

Radeck, W. (2008d) Analytical methods for the determination of ractopamine in different matrices. Meeting of the WG on Ractopamine, Panel of Additives and Products used in Animal Feed (FEEDAP), EFSA.

Radeck, W. (2008e) Analytik von pharmakologisch wirksamen Stoffen mittels LC-MS/MS. Analytica, München 2008.

Stoyke, M. (2008a) Evaluation of NRCP – Substance group: B2e. CRL-Workshop 2008, Berlin, 03 to 06 June 2008.

Stoyke, M. (2008b) Evaluation of Interlaboratory Study NIIM_09/07. CRL-Workshop 2008, Berlin, 03 to 06 June 2008.

Stoyke, M. (2008c) Follow-up Measures. CRL-Workshop 2008, Berlin, 03 to 06 June 2008.

Stoyke, M. (2008d) Assessment of Homogeneity and Calculation of Combination Scores. CRL-Workshop 2008, Berlin, 03 to 06 June 2008.

Stoyke, M. (2008e) Auswertung der Laborvergleichsuntersuchung – Nitroimidazole in Ei – NIIM_09/07. NRL Fachtagung 2008, Berlin, 17 to 18 June 2008.

Stoyke, M. (2008f) Auswertung Laborvergleichsstudie Anthelmintika in Milch - ANTH_04/08. NRL Fachtagung 2008, Berlin, 17 to 18 June 2008.

4.9
Staff of the CRL Berlin

4.9.1 Management

P. Gowik	Director of the CRL Berlin (not financed by the EC)
J. Polzer	Deputy Director (not financed by the EC)

4.9.2 Analytical Services

W. Radeck	Senior Scientist, Head of HPLC division
J. Polzer	Senior Scientist, Head of GC-Division, Quality Manager of Group 5 "Analyses" (not financed by the EC)
M. Stoyke	Scientist, HPLC division, proficiency test organisation, evaluation
F. Hamann	Senior Scientist, Animal Studies
C. Bieber	Technician
B. Matthes	Technician (66.6%)
S. Maidhof	Technician (66.6%)
M. Schramm	Technician (11.7%) until 15 January 08

4.9.3 Administration, Documentation, Translation

M. Jüsgen	Translator (88.3%)

4.10 Organigram of the CRL Berlin

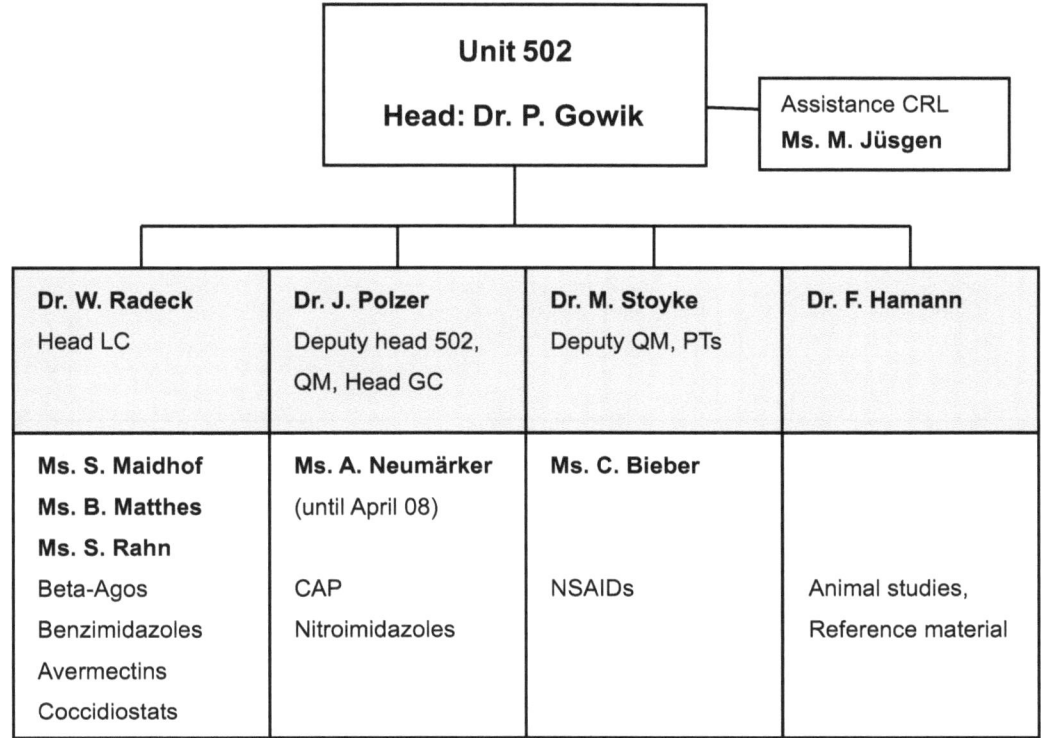

5 Breakdown of personnel and financial capacities (Annex)

5.1
General Tasks

sub items		share of staff time [d]	share % of total staff time	staff costs	staff costs % of total budget	consumables costs	consumables % of total budget
1.	Meeting 4 CRLs; EC-4 CRL for residues management[a]	1	0.1	356 €	0.1	0 €	0.0
2.	EC/CRL related EC and International Bodies; Co-operation with international organisations[b]	20	1.4	7,119 €	1.6	0 €	0.0
3.	Reports, cost estimate, documentation[c]	104.3	7.5	34,145 €	7.6	0 €	0.0
sum		125.3	9.0	41,621 €	9.3	0 €	0.0

[a] yearly task, meeting at EuroResidue VI. It was an extra meeting with the 3 CRLs concerned. The CRL attended with two colleagues. Some work had to be carried in preparation of this meeting and afterwards. Therefore 1 working day was counted for this meeting.
[b] yearly task Codex MRLs, CCRVDF CCMAS, BIPM, CEN/ISO, IRMM.
[c] yearly task evaluation NRCPs, work plan, cost estimate, technical report, financial report, interim report.

5.2
Development and Validation of Analytical Methods and Animal Studies[1]

	sub items	share of staff time [d]	share % of total staff time	staff costs	staff costs % of total budget	consumables costs	consumables % of total budget
1.	Investigation of distribution / depletion of nitroimidazoles in hens[a]	81	5.8	24,401 €	5.4	0 €	0.0
2.	Development and validation of method for beta-agonists in hair and urine by LC-MSMS[b]	75	5.4	22,950 €	5.1	0 €	0.0
3.	Validation of method for beta-agonists in retina by LC-MSMS[c]	56	4.0	14,878 €	3.3	0 €	0.0
4.	Optimisation and validation of a method for avermectins in aquaculture[d]	116	8.3	30,616 €	6.8	0 €	0.0
5.	Long-term stability studies for all substance groups[e]	77	5.5	19,916 €	4.4	0 €	0.0
6.	Research and identification of unknown compounds[f]	3	0.2	943 €	0.2	0 €	0.0
sum		408	29.3	113,704 €	25.4	0 €	0.0

[a] finished within reference period depletion study in muscle and eggs There was a mistake in the interim report. The animal study was finalised but not the measurements. Only a part of the analytes/samples were analysed until end of July. In addition the studies included new analytes (Tinidazol and Carnidazol) which had never been analysed before. So additionally some technical analytical problems (e.g. with the application of Q-TOF measurements which became necessary for the elucidation of possible metabolites) had to be overcome which lead to this high number of working days.
[b] Hair method could not be validated because of difficulties in the development of the method.
[c] finished within reference period agreed upon with COM.
[d] finished within reference period.
[e] yearly task.
[f] yearly task.

[1] Annex V, chapter 2, section 1 (a, c, d)

5.3
Quality assurance and quality control including the development of incurred test material and the organisation of a proficiency test (22 %)[2]

sub items		share of staff time [d]	share % of total staff time	staff costs	staff costs % of total budget	consumables costs	consumables % of total budget
1.	Maintenance of equipment, documentation, audits, management[a]	131	9.4	39,979 €	8.9	0 €	0.0
2.	Proficiency test on benzimidazoles in milk: characterisation of the material, packaging, evaluation[b]	150	10.8	43,765 €	9.8	0 €	0.0
3.	Cooperation with IRMM for the production of CRM for nitroimidazoles[c]	31	2.2	9,041 €	2.0	0 €	0.0
4.	Production of incurred sample material; treatments of aquaculture (avermectins); hens with nitroimidazoles; beta-agonists in cattle hair and urine[d]	70	5.0	19,740 €	4.4	0 €	0.0
sum		382	27.5	112,524 €	25.1	0 €	0.0

[a] yearly task.
[b] finished within reference period. During the second half of 2008 the report had to be written and an extensive and work intensive evaluation of the data started. So additionally 50 working days of a scientist were needed to finalise the report. The preparation of the proficiency test, i.e. material production, homogeneity and stability testing, shipping, documentation etc. is a mixed work of scientist and technical assistants (TA) and therefore also a mixed calculation of the staff costs. TAs earn less money than scientists therefore more working days result for less costs.
[c] Finalized. Here a difference to the IR occurs. This was most probably a "mistake" in the IR since the IR can only be an estimation. The FR is the one which has to be the correct one. So please take the figure of the FR as the correct one.
[d] to be finished within reference period avermectins: for the production of reference material nitroimidazoles: in 2006 only eggs were produced; for further knowledge of behaviour in muscle new hens have to be treated to be compared with results from turkey beta-agonists: production of reference material when sufficient in amount and concentration and when homogeneity can be achieved; to be used for a PT in 2009

---

[2] Annex V, chapter 2, section 1 (a, b, c, g)

5.4
Technical and scientific support to Member States, the Commission, including arbitration and training activities (44 %)[3]

	sub items	share of staff time [d]	share % of total staff time	staff costs	staff costs % of total budget	consumables costs	consumables % of total budget
1.	Technical, scientific support and training[a]	215	15.5	70,990 €	15.8	0 €	0.0
2.	follow-up of PT[b]	5	0.4	1,719 €	0.4	0 €	0.0
3.	Provision of standard substances incl. procuring, storage, administration, documentation, shipment etc.[c]	134	9.6	39,745 €	8.9	0 €	0.0
4.	Analysis of official samples[d]	47	3.4	13,052 €	2.9	0 €	0.0
5.	Visit of NRLs[e]	15	1.1	5,158 €	1.2	0 €	0.0
6.	Organisation and performance of a workshop[f]	60	4.3	17,920 €	4.0	0 €	0.0
sum		476	34.2	148,585 €	33.2	0 €	0.0
	Total	1,391.3	100.0	416,434 €	92.9	0 €	0.0

[a] yearly task. During the first half of 2008 we were very busy with the preparation and performance of the workshop, the participation (2 oral presentations and 6 posters, papers for proceedings) at EURORESIDUE VI and the preparation of the proficiency test. Therefore less time was left for other tasks like support and training. This changed in the second half.
[b] necessary working time depends on request for follow-up measures. Here a difference to the IR occurs. This was most probably a "mistake" in the IR since the IR can only be an estimation. The FR is the one which has to be the correct one. So please take the figure of the FR as the correct one.
[c] yearly task.
[d] 32 official samples were analysed for confirmatory purposes. Some samples arrive as single samples. But sometimes we get two or more samples at once which then reduce the time needed for analyses. Secondly, different matrices require different methods and therefore different time for their analyses. Therefore the time for 47 samples is not in congruency with the time for 19 samples.
[e] The NRL in Budapest/Hungary was visited.
[f] yearly task. Reduction in comparison to IR. Other tasks like the investigation of the nitroimidazole samples or the development and establishment of the hair method, technical support etc required so much time that it would have surpassed 100% working time for the scientists (which indeed they did but what cannot be reported officially). So I had to reduce the necessary time for another task. Nevertheless the work was done.

---
[3] Annex V, chapter 2, section 1 (d, f, h, l)

MIX
Papier aus verantwortungsvollen Quellen
Paper from responsible sources
FSC® C105338

If you have any concerns about our products,
you can contact us on
ProductSafety@springernature.com
In case Publisher is established outside the EU,
the EU authorized representative is:
Springer Nature Customer Service Center GmbH
Europaplatz 3, 69115 Heidelberg, Germany

Printed by Libri Plureos GmbH
in Hamburg, Germany